Essential Oils

By SSS

Using Essential Oils For An All Natural Solution To Laundry Needs With No Chemicals & Toxins

Table of Contents

Introduction

As trivial as it may appear, keeping your clothes clean and maintaining their color is one of the most commonly encountered issues in any household. Though there are many detergents available in the market that claim to keep the 'newness' of your clothes intact, more often than not, they hamper the clothes in a negative manner.

A good thing nowadays is that people are extremely cautious about the ingredients that are used in the products they directly use. The major issue with detergents is they contain many harsh chemicals. These chemicals affect the quality of clothes and eventually the fabric becomes dull and weak. The chemicals are also harmful which may cling to the skin and cause allergic reactions or skin rashes.

Due to this, toxic chemical laced products are getting replaced with greener solutions that are clothes, skin and health friendly.

Another issue in regards with laundry is related to drying of clothes. Most of us use driers, but the clothes suffer from static cling wherein the fabric creates friction against each other and the quality of clothes gets further damaged. Wool dryer balls were invented to solve this issue and they gave good results.

Thus we see that even though continuous research is going on in the laundry industry, new challenges are coming up now and then. The above mentioned laundry problems are very common but diverse in nature. Is there a common solution to these problems?

Of course, there is and this book is going to introduce this miracle to you i.e. essential oils. Essential oils are a gift of nature which has many applications ranging from medicinal value to cosmetic benefits.

In this book we will learn about what essential oils offer in the field of laundry cleaning. I have also discussed the benefits of using essential oils over commercial laundry cleaning products, which will help you make the right decision for you and your family. The book also contains the recipes which contain essential oils for various laundry needs like washing clothes, softening them and drying them.

I want to thank you for choosing this book and I hope you enjoy reading the book and use the recipes mentioned for your laundry.

Let's get started!

Chapter 1: What Are Essential Oils?

Essential oils are oils that are derived from the various parts of plants. They are all natural and not adulterated with mineral oil or any artificial compound. While the normal oils are derived mainly from plant seeds, for example almond and peanut oil; essential oils are derived from other parts of the plant. They are volatile in nature and have a distinct aroma because of the aromatic compounds present in them. Unlike normal oils, they are non greasy and are highly concentrated in nature.

Essential oils have various uses owing to their unique chemical properties. Mostly because of their distinctive smell, they are used in cosmetics and perfumes. They are also used by some alternative medicine practitioners in aromatherapy.

It is believed that essential oils can diffuse easily in human body and can help it relax. It also has mind relaxing properties and is often used in various types of massages. Some essential oils are used for the treatment of cold and cough too. Few essential oils have been used from a long time as antiseptics.

There are various types of essential oils. They can vary from each other in their properties, the source of extraction and applications. I have discussed some common properties of these essential oils. Pay attention to the properties of these oils and use them in your laundry as you need or deem correct for your family and your good health.

Lemongrass:

Distilled from an Asian tropical grass, it is called so because of its strong lemony smell. It is commonly found in room fresheners, insect repellants, soaps and detergents. This essential oil is perfect to get sweaty odors off of your clothes. However, it is important to know how much needs to be used in order to make the best use of it. The smell can be quite strong and is also said to repel insects. Many trekkers and others who savor outdoor sports prefer to soak their clothes in lemon grass concoctions in order to repel insects such as fleas and ticks.

Tea Tree:

Derived from tea leaves, this oil is spicy and warm in nature. It is often used in combination with other essential oils like rosemary or nutmeg. It is used to make colognes and aftershaves with spicy scent. It is also used in aromatherapy for its purifying and uplifting affects on the body. Tea tree oil is also used in skin creams and ointments. This is perfect for people who are hounded by body odor, as clothes that smell of tea tree oil will help ward of the stench of sweat, or rather mute it. Again, the strong flavor is something that needs to be used with caution. Some prefer to soak their clothes in this oil if they suffer from body acne as it is scientifically proven that tea tree helps in killing acne causing bacteria and prevents rashes.

Pine:

It is prepared by the distillation of needles and branches of the Scotch pine tree, which grows in Asia and Europe. It smells like resin and wood. It is one of the most preferred household scents. It can help open the pores of skin and tone it. But it should be used in small quantities on the skin or it can cause a burning sensation to the skin. Perfect for those who are allergic to commercial cleaning products as this can help in soothing the skin without aggravating the condition. Using this oil to wash clothes will make them smell woody and help keep body odor at bay.

Rose Otto:

Distilled from rose petals, this is one of the most sought after essential oil. It has got a warm, intense and a rich rosy smell. It can uplift your mood and make the surroundings more romantic. It has a calming and luxurious feel to it, so it is often used in massages. The oil is also used in powders, skin creams and body lotions. Use it as a relaxant in your laundry, as your clothes will smell great and lift your mood. It is not a bad idea to use this and soak your table cloth in and help your dining room smell pleasant. The same extends to your bed spreads and will help your bedrooms smell pleasant and relax you completely.

Ylang Ylang:

This oil is distilled from the flowers of Cananga tree. It is made sure that the flowers are picked up early in the morning as it affects the quality of the oil. The distillation process is broken down into several steps and the accumulated oil is separated at each level. The oil collected first is of the highest grade and is called "Ylang Ylang Extra". It has an intense sweet scent, which is very floral and it helps stimulate the senses and creates a mood of euphoria. Consider using this if you wish to come across as a person with a strong personality as you will reek of amazing and exciting freshness if you use this oil for washing your clothes.

Nutmeg:

Nutmegs are spices that are extensively grown in Asia. They have a woody smell and look pretty. Nutmegs are cut into small pieces and pressed first to remove the fixed oil called as nutmeg butter. The pieces are then dried and distilled to obtain the nutmeg essential oil. It has a spicy and oily scent and is a major component in men's perfumes. The woody smell that it imparts is said to help men reel under a sense of delight. And oh, it is popular amongst women too! The effects are revitalizing and mood uplifting. Who needs expensive perfume when your clothes smell of nutmeg oil?

Myrrh:

One of the oldest essential oils, myrrh has been present since the ancient Egyptian civilization. It has a unique balsamic spicy aroma which heats up the body. It is preferred to be used in combination with woody scent perfumes. It is also used in skin creams and ointments. In ancient Egypt it was used for embalming dead bodies so that they wouldn't rot easily. Subsequently they would be mummified and several mummies that were recently uncovered were all in near perfect condition. So if you wish your clothes to remain new for long then consider washing them with a little myrrh. It has a revitalizing and meditative effect. Myrrh is a great addition to your organic laundry solution.

Lemon:

Lemon essential oil can be obtained from distilling lemon peels or cold pressing them. The fragrance is a fresh one and instantly tickles the senses. Just a small whiff is enough to enliven a person and cause him or her to wake up. It is used frequently in body bath shampoos and massage oils. Lemon oil is also preferred to be used as room fresheners and bathroom fragrances. It is also used in deodorants to mask the body odor, especially in tropical countries where the level of sweating is simply high.

Citronella:

Two types of citronella essential oils are available, Java type and Ceylon type. Citronella has a warm, woody, grassy smell. Hence, it is preferred a lot as an outdoor freshener and for room and furniture sprays. Java citronella oil is produced in many parts of the world but Ceylon citronella plant is specifically grown in Sri Lanka. Java oil tends to be more on the floral, sweeter side so it is preferred in perfumes. It has a purifying and rejuvenating fragrance. Citronella is said to be the number 1 mosquito repellant oil that most commercial repellants use in their preparations.

Mosquitoes will drop dead just by smelling the scent from afar. Many trekkers and outdoor sports enthusiasts carry some citronella essential oil with them to mask their body odor and prevent mosquitoes, ticks and leeches from adhering to their bodies.

Eucalyptus:

Eucalyptus essential oil is primarily derived from *Eucalyptus globules*. It has medicinal properties and is used in traditional medicines. It is used to relieve muscle pain and stiffness. It is also applied on wounds to make them less painful. It has a purifying and reviving effect. Use this essential oil in your laundry to ward off cold and blocked nose. You can consider dipping your hanky in a bowl of water containing a couple of drops of the oil and using it to place over your nose. Your sinus will release and you will be able to breathe properly once more.

Palmarosa:

It is distilled from Palmarosa grass which is closely related to citronella and lemon grass. It has a floral yet grassy scent and is therefore very helpful in distressing the mind and body. It is also used to tone the skin and helps to prevent wrinkles. It is also a component of bath and massage oils. Many people prefer to use this with their house clothes as it helps them remain fresh and feel rejuvenated.

Myrtle:

This oil is distilled from the myrtle plant found in the Mediterranean region. It has spicy camphor like aroma. Better grade myrtle oils tend to be sweeter and fresh smelling. It is used as a room freshener and in mens colognes. In combination with lavender, rosemary, bergamot, clary sage and lime oils it can produce a very good fragrance, which is mostly used in luxury perfumes. So this is best used with clothes that you would wear to important meetings and events and can also be a good scent to try for high tea events.

Geranium:

Geranium oil is extracted from the leaves and flowers of the geranium plant. The scent is sweet smelling and is said to be quite strong. Many people use this essential oil to render a sweet fragrance to their detergents and in turn, their clothes. The oil has the property of closing open pores so it is ideal for people that have an oily skin to use. Its astringent properties protect the clothes from losing lint.

Sweet orange:

Sweet orange extract is probably the most widely used essential oil in the world. It is quite cheap and easy to prepare. Its sweet fragrance helps in adding a sweet flavor to detergents. Sweet orange is also skin friendly and the oil has the tendency to loosen dirt and tough stains. So it is ideal to use this in combination to other essential oils and can also be used independently to prepare sweet smelling detergents.

Lavender:

Who in this world is not familiar with the sweet smell of lavender? Lavender essential oil is extracted from lavender flowers and it is used in a wide variety of commercial products including room fresheners, toilet fresheners, soaps, toiletries, pot Pourri etc. You can use this oil to add to your detergents and help your clothes smell fresh.

Basil:

Basil essential oil is a good choice for detergents. The smell of basil is said to help people calm down. It also aids in better blood circulation and so, soaking your clothes in it will help you remain healthy. It is also extremely mild on the skin and will help in preventing eye irritation.

Peppermint:

Peppermint essential oil is known for its antiseptic and anti bacterial properties. The oil is ideal for those who sweat a lot and will completely get rid of germs present on clothes. You can use just a few drops for a large pile of clothes. It is best to use if you are a sports person.

Chapter 2: Essential Oils And Laundry

We discussed the challenges faced while doing laundry at the start of the book. Fortunately, Essential oils offer a good solution to laundry related problems, as these oils can be used as detergents, fabric softeners and also drying agents. The cleaning solutions made from essential oils don't contain harmful chemicals present in conventional detergents and helps maintain the quality of the clothes.

Essential oils in Detergents

Conventional laundry detergents contain chemicals like EDTA, chlorine bleach and phosphate which damage our health. Most of the skin allergies and rashes are primarily caused by these damaging agents. In fact, several chemicals that are used in detergents are not even fully approved and a lot of them are not supposed to be used at all. There has been many a crackdown where detergents were tested and chemicals that cause skin and other problems were identified. Grownups have the capacity to cope but imagine what would happen to poor children's sensitive skin. So the best solution is to shift to natural ingredients, which will be slightly mellow on the skin and not cause any internal damage. These alternatives are essential oils.

Apart from protecting us from the harmful effects of chemical detergents, essential oils also provide an array of other benefits. As discussed earlier, essential oils have aromatherapy properties owing to their aromatic chemical structure. Because of their unique chemical structure, they help in maintaining the well being of our body as well as our mind. Many essential oils are known to have de-stressing properties. Clothes that have essence of such essential oils relax people and keep them more refreshed. The mind becomes stimulated resulting in an increased productivity yet remains calm to take important decisions. The body feels more energetic and less fatigued. Therefore, with increasing age it is suggested to use essential oils in our day to day lives. Essential oils also protect the fabric of clothes for a longer duration. Apart from adding a new shine, good smell and freshness to our clothes; they can also act as insect repellants. Peppermint, spearmint, citronella, catnip and lemongrass are known to repel insects. Adding them to the laundry protects the clothes from insect attacks, especially when the clothes need to be stored for a long time like heavy woolen clothes. People who live in tropical areas are also very susceptible to insect attacks and their clothes get dirty easily. In such cases, essential oils should be added to detergent. Basil has strong mosquito repellant properties. So people who live in mosquito prone areas should regularly use basil essential oil in their laundry mix. Instead of opting for chemical mosquito repellants which are applied directly on skin and can harm it, why not to make our clothes mosquito repellent by all natural means?

Essential oils are an all organic solution to this problem and they can easily replace the commercially available detergents. Various essential oils have various roles in laundry industry, while choosing the oil for your detergent, refer to the following table:

Chamomile	Soothes the skin
Lavender	Relaxes the muscle
Peppermint, Eucalyptus	Protects against cold and sinus
Rosemary	Calms the senses
Cedar	Gives a woody clean scent
Lemon	Whitens cloth and adds shine to them, also stimulates senses
Tea Tree	Anti bacterial and anti fungal
Sweet orange	Removes stains and whitens laundry

These essential oils can be added directly to your detergents if you don't want to prepare the detergent from scratch. It is advisable to use organic detergents or laundry products as opposed to your chemical laden commercial detergents, when you mix them essential oils. Organic detergent will not cause any damage to your clothes or your body, and the addition of the essential oils will add their beneficial properties. They are prepared from olive extracts and do not contain LYE. You can buy them in bulk if you wish to save money.

Few essential oil that can be added to your organic detergents are Lavender, Lemongrass, Citrus fresh and Eucalyptus. Their properties and usefulness was discussed in detail in the previous chapter.

Adding them to your detergent will help you get the best of both worlds; the benefits of essential oil and the cleaning of your organic detergent. However, the essential oils scent won't be noticeable in the strong presence of the components of your detergent. About 3 to 5 drops of the oil can be directly added to the wash cycle, or a tablespoon can be added beforehand to the detergent. You can pre measure a few drops or get yourself a dropper to help you out. It is a good idea to have small cups that you can use to measure out the essential oils individually.

If you are using two or more different ones then remember that you have to think if they will go well together. There can be a few strong scented ones such as nutmeg and myrtle which might not go well together. You might have to do a little trial and error before knowing which combination works best.

Essential oil can also be used to prepare detergent for your clothes. These detergents can be completely prepared at your home using easy recipes. Though the recipes contain the use of washing soda, which is a chemical, the quantity and the procedure is varied in such a way that the harmful effects are minimized drastically. The recipes remain more or less same in nature with the difference in the quantity of the additives. So you can prepare them in bulk and store them in plastic jars and use them as you would normal detergent. If you fear them losing their aroma then considering storing the excess in Ziploc bags to ensure preserving the scent.

Here are few of the recipes discussed:

Basic Borax Laundry Solution

Materials Required:

- 2 cups borax
- 2 cups bar soap (grated)
- 2 cups washing soda
- 1 liter of boiling water
- one tablespoon of essential oil of choice

Procedure:

1. Boil the water on low heat.
2. Add the grated soap bar slowly and keep stirring till it has completely melted and there are no lumps left.
3. Add a teaspoon of the essential oil you desire.
4. Pour the liquid mixture into a large bucket (make sure it is pretty big)
5. Add borax and washing soda.
6. Add 2 gallons of water and mix the whole concoction till everything is uniform.
7. Use ¼th cup for every wash load. Stir the mixture before using it as it can start to set.

Glycerin Laundry Solution for Sensitive Skin
Materials Required:

- ½ cup of borax
- 6 cups of water
- 2 pints of hot water
- 1/3rd bar of grated Fels-Naphtha
- ½ cup of washing soda
- 2 tablespoons of glycerin

Procedure:

1. Mix the grated Fels-Naphtha soap in 6 cups of water properly.
2. Heat this mixture on low heat till everything becomes a homogenous blend.
3. Add a teaspoon of essential oil of your choice.
4. Add borax and washing soda.
5. Stir the mixture till it thickens and the remove from heat.
6. Pour two pints of hot water in a large bucket.
7. Pour the soap mixture in this bucket and add glycerin.
8. Mix the blend well and set it aside for 24 hours so that it is gelled completely.
9. After 24 hours, add hot water to the mixture till it liquefies again and use it in your wash load.

All Natural Organic Laundry Solution
The below given recipe is an all natural recipe for preparing laundry soap. This recipe doesn't include washing soda and it ideal for those who are allergic to washing soda. This all natural recipe will have no side effects on the skin or the cloth

whatsoever. It can be used for any laundry but is mostly preferred for cotton linens and clothes that are dried naturally.

Materials Required:

- ½ cup aloe vera juice
- 1 cup water
- ½ cup white vinegar
- 2 cups organic liquid castile soap
- 1 tablespoon citric acid powder
- 2 tablespoons grapefruit seed extract
- 15 to 20 drops of essential oil

Procedure:

1. Mix all the ingredients in a container. They can be mixed in any order.
2. Shake the container well; turn it upside down at least once or twice.
3. Use 1/4th cup to add in a wash load.

Laundry Solution for Delicate Clothing

The below recipe is most suitable for delicate clothing items like lingerie and knit wear. But avoid using it on hundred percent satin, wool and silk material.

Material Required:

- 1 cup rosemary mixture
- 1 ounce liquid castile soap

Procedure:

1. Add 2 twigs of bruised rosemary or 1 teaspoon of dried and crushed rosemary or 3 drops of rosemary essential oil to a cup of boiling water.

2. Load your clothes in the washer and pour liquid castile soap and rosemary infusion into the washer.
3. Set the washer on gentle cycle using cold water.

Rejuvenating Laundry Solution
Materials Required

- one cup of borax
- one bar of natural organic detergent or soap
- one cup of washing soda
- twenty drops of lemon essential oil

Procedure

1. Grate the soap bar into fine particles. Make sure the particles are very small for easy dissolution.
2. Mix the borax and the washing soda with the grated bar.
3. Once the concoction is ready, add lemon essential oil to it and make sure it is distributed uniformly.
4. Store in an air tight container.
5. Use one to two tablespoons per load.

Various essential oil blends can be used to clean laundry instead of one essential oil. Here few combinations are given which are tried and tested and gave good results.

Tea Tree Essential oil blend:

- 40 drops of tea tree
- 30 drops of lemongrass or lemon
- 20 drops of Palmarosa
- Lavender essential oil blend
- 40 drops of lavender

- 30 drops of lemongrass or lemon
- 20 drops of clove

Citrus essential oil blend
- 30 drops of orange
- 30 drops of grapefruit
- 30 drops of lemongrass or lime

Essential oils in fabric softeners

Fabric softeners were devised as a method to combat the harsh detergents and their after effects on clothes. Commercial fabric softeners contain a huge amount of toxic materials and also artificial fragrances to mask the odor of chemicals. They contain chemicals like Benzyl alcohol (which causes upper respiratory tract irritant), Ethyl acetate (classified narcotic on EPA's hazardous waste list), benzyl acetate (can cause pancreatic cancer), camphor (can disturb central nervous system) etc. So essential oils have emerged as an alternative. Few of the recipes are given below which make use of essential oil as fabric softeners:

Au Natural Fabric Softener
Materials Required:

- One cup distilled white vinegar
- Half tablespoon essential oil (any oil of your choice)

Procedure:

1. Mix one cup distilled white vinegar and half tablespoon essential oil of your choice.
2. Once the concoction is prepared, fill a spray bottle with it.

3. Shake it well and spray on the clothes at least ten times before you put your clothes in dryer.

Important point: Use an essential oil that has a strong scent which can completely mask the smell of vinegar. Eucalyptus oil is one of the most preferred options.

Protecting Clothes against Acidic Substance
The following recipe is an alkaline nature fabric softener which can reverse the effects of acid attacks on your clothes.

Materials Required:

- Half cup baking soda
- Two cups of Epsom salt or course sea salt
- 20 to 30 drops of essential oil of your choice

Procedure:

1. Mix two cups of Epsom salt with essential oil till the oil is evenly distributed in the salt mixture.
2. Add half a cup of baking soda to the concoction.
3. Pour them in a container.
4. Add two to three tablespoons of this mixture to your clothes while giving them the final rinse after washing.

Chapter 3: Wool Dryer Balls

A special segment is dedicated to wool dryer balls, as these make great laundry dryers when used with essential oils. They typically consist of wool balls that bounce in the dryer, circulating the whole area so that there are enough gaps present between clothes for hot air circulation. They reduce wrinkles and fluff in the laundry. Plastic dryer balls should be avoided as they release chemicals when heated. Only all natural wool dryer balls should be used.

Below mentioned are some of the benefits of using a wool dryer ball

> ➢ They absorb the extra moisture from your clothes and help them dry fast.
> ➢ They are better compared to dryer sheets and fabric softeners, as they don't contain chemicals. So the clothes are chemical free and our skin is also protected.
> ➢ Dryer sheets are costly and can't be reused. On the other hand, wool dryer balls can be used for years without any change in efficiency and you don't have to worry about running out of them when you have to dry something important.
> ➢ After a point commercial softeners can reduce the absorbing efficiency of towels, diapers and kitchen cloths and force you to buy new ones even if they are fairly new. But wool dryers won't affect it no matter how many times they are dried.
> ➢ Commercial softeners can't be used on every type of cloth. It is specially warned to never use them on baby clothes as the chemicals can be extremely dangerous and cause sensitive baby skin to erupt into rashes. Wool dryers are suitable for

clothes of any type as it is made from natural materials and is completely safe for all clothes including baby's clothes.

> They reduce static cling hundred percent, which is one of the biggest problems for clothes that are dried in an electronic dryer. So you don't have to worry about your synthetic clothes causing friction and giving you mini shocks or your hair standing up just because you are wearing a polyester top.

> All your dryer related problems will be solved when you decide to use wool dryer balls to dry your clothes.

How to make your own Wool dryer Balls?

Choosing the material - Make sure you opt for hundred percent wool yarns. There should be no blend in the yarn, like acrylic blend yarn. There are many types of wool yarns available in the market; the most preferred one is lightly spun, thick roving yarn. Instead of buying a yarn, you can undo an old woolen sweater. You can also choose a muffler or your baby's woolens which he or she has outgrown. Basically, any old woolen that is no longer of use to you can be repurposed to make wool dryer balls.

Important tip: Avoid "machine washable" and "super wash" wool yarn. This type will not felt and thus will not absorb the moisture properly. They can also open up inside the dryer lead to a mess. You can either choose colored wool balls or uncolored ones. Colored balls are easy to identify and separate from the pile of clothes but be careful while choosing them. The yarn shouldn't bleed and spoil the rest of the load.

Other materials which are required:

> Scissors
> blunt tipped needle
> pantyhose and a cotton string (don't use a wool string or it will fluff outside the final structure)

Procedure

1. Start wrapping the yarn around your two figures for a minimum of two minutes.
2. Pinch and secure this bundle of yarn and start wrapping a second round of yarn around this preformed bundle.
3. After a few rounds, you'll notice the beginning of the ball. Keep wrapping till the whole ball is formed in a desires size (You can make balls ranging from tennis balls to baseball balls).
4. Use the blunt tipped needle to tuck the remaining thread inside the yarn ball. Pull the last remaining thread through the yarn ball and cut it.
5. Cut one of the legs from the pantyhose and put the ball inside it. Secure the whole structure using the cotton thread.

How to use Wool dryer balls?

A prerequisite to using wool dryer balls is that they should be felted. Felting occurs when the wool strands don't separate on scraping with fingers. Felted wool balls should be used otherwise its strands might get loose in the. To felt the balls, throw the entire batch of ball into a load of towels. Wash the load in hot wash cycle but rinse it in cold water rinse cycle. Set the dryer to the hottest drying setting and dry the batch. Remove the pantyhose and check the balls for felting. You may require repeating this procedure three to four times as not all wool yarn will felt in the first try itself.

As was said earlier, using colored balls will help you identify them better but white ones will allow you to eliminate doubt of bleeding. You must try and check if the ball is bleeding by using white towels for the felting process. If the towels have changed color then it is best to discard the batch and choose colorless ones to avoid the problem from repeating.

Once the balls are felted, they should look like tennis balls and not have any lose threads on them. They should be smooth and slightly hard.

To use the felted balls, just throw them along with your laundry in the dryer. For average loads, at least four balls should be used to decrease the drying duration. For large loads, minimum six balls should be used. The dryer balls can be stored in the dryer itself after the completion of the procedure but make sure you keep the door of the dryer open in order for any odor to escape and excess water to dry off completely before using it again.

Essential oils and wool dryer balls

Essential oils can penetrate into the fabric well when drying the clothes. Since the fiber strands are exposed to hot air and wool dryer balls, essential oils can easily seep into the clothes and also remain on them for a longer duration. Hence, to make maximum use of essential oils in the laundry, add them to the wool dryer balls. Just put two to three drops of the oil on each ball and toss them in your dryer. The essential oils can last up to the three cycles in the dryer before their affects start to fade. Various combinations of oil can be used here:

- ➤ For sheets and towels, 2 balls of peppermint and two balls of ylang-ylang could be used.
- ➤ If you perspire a lot, two balls of lemon and two balls of lavender can be used for those cotton shirts!
- ➤ 2 balls of rose Otto and two balls of Palmarosa will work great if you have a date or party to attend.

Precautions while handling essential oils

As beneficial as they are, essential oils also come with a lot of risks. They are natural products so they don't pose hazards like chemicals and synthetic materials, but they still require a lot of care while handling, especially when using them as raw material for preparing laundry formulations. Some of the risks associated with them along with the precautions are listed below and it is best that you observe these in order to keep your clothes and yourself safe

Essential oils are highly concentrated in nature. 250 pounds of peppermint leaves are used to prepare 1 pound of essential oil. Similarly, 150 pounds of lavender flowers are used to prepare 1 pound of essential oil. In preparation of 1 pound of rose essential oil, thousands of pounds of roses are used!! So be very careful while using them. Just a small drop will help you avail the benefit and scent of a large load of the base ingredient. Many people don't realize this and end up using the oils in excess. Make sure you make use of the measures that are mentioned in this book and do not use any more than that.

Remember that less is more with essential oils. So don't be tempted to add in a little extra just because you are not getting the desired smell. It is easy to get carried away and before you know it, you are forced to discard the batch because of a pungent fragrance thanks to over adding the oils. So make sure you exercise precaution when using the oils and only add how much ever is needed to make the detergent. If you are directly adding then it is best to dilute the oil and thin it down before adding to your machine.

Since essential oils are directly derived from their plant parts, they contain the properties of the plant in the most concentrated form. Menthol herb gives a cooling tingling sensation on tongue. But if menthol essential oil is consumed directly, the tongue will be stimulated in excess which can actually cause burning sensation and pain. Similarly, excess menthol in your clothes might make you uncomfortable. You might feel extremely uneasy and might have to get out of your clothes to wash them and get into new ones. So use the strong scented oils sparingly and make sure they are not used on baby clothes as he or she might feel uncomfortable.

Essential oils should never be applied on skin in undiluted forms. They have small molecular size so they can enter and circulate the body easily. Skin can have allergic reactions and it can also result in development of permanent hypersensitivity to the oil. When you are using essential oil to prepare any of the laundry concoctions, use them in a diluted form. If you are using them undiluted for better results, wear gloves while handling their bottles or containers and don't touch your face while working with it. You will have to buy good quality gloves that are thick enough and do not allow oils to permeate through. Keep them away from your other clothes as they might give off a strong odor.

Apart from gloves, you need to use other safety equipment if necessary including goggles and full sleeve shirts. If you are getting your kids to help out then keep an eye on them and make sure that they are also appropriately dressed for the occasion. Always use a glass bowl or a ceramic one to prepare as some oils and detergent chemicals can have a reaction on plastic. You might end up creating invisible fumes that can be dangerous to you and your family members. Make sure you do not use the same bowls for the next batch unless it is thoroughly cleaned and sterilized and don't use it for food preparations.

Even the smell of concentrated essential oil is enough to give some people headaches. While testing out new oils for your laundry first open the bottle cap partially and check if you feel any kind of unease in its presence. If you feel dizziness or your senses tickle too much, it is best to avoid the particular essential oil. If you don't wish to waste them then consider testing them at the store itself. Ask the helper to open it and allow you to smell it before you purchase. You can also get a little applied to your skin to test if it is okay to be used on your skin.

Even while putting them in detergent formulations or wool dryer balls, don't exceed the amount mentioned in the procedure. The oil is going to penetrate your clothes and will also come in contact with your skin. Over usage of the oil can turn your own clothes hazardous if you are sensitive to these oils.

Some essential oils can make your skin more photosensitive in nature. If you use any citrus based essential oils like orange, lemon, grapefruit, and lime, be sure not to expose yourself in direct sunlight. It can lead to rashes, discoloration of the skin or blisters. So it is a good idea to not use these on your beach ware as they might have an effect on the parts of your body which they come in contact with. Just make sure that you don't use these on your children's uniforms as well as they might have to spend time in the sun playing.

During pregnancy take extra precautions while using essential oils for your laundry. They can cross the placenta and reach the baby. Even a slight high quantity of essential oil can damage your unborn baby's health drastically, even if it doesn't affect you much. If possible, avoid using essential oils when pregnant. If you still want to use them, take essential oil based aromatherapy massages and make sure to use diluted concoctions.

Aniseed, Angelica, Mustard, Jasmine, Marjoram, Clary Sage, clove, myrrh, fennel, thyme, basil, black pepper, chamomile, cinnamon, peppermint, wintergreen fir, horseradish and ginger should be consumed in a very less quantity or should not be consumed at all during pregnancy.

Remember to keep your essential oils away from open flames. They can be inflammable and some are also volatile and may catch fire at any time. Do not have you lab situated inside the kitchen as it is extremely dangerous. Make sure you do not place the bottles near a fire place as all of them might spontaneously catch fire. Try and remain as careful as possible especially if you have young children and pets in your house.

Some essential oils are not suitable for people suffering from respiratory problems such as asthma and bronchitis. If you wish to use an essential oil then it is best to consult a physician first. He or she will guide you and suggest the best oil that can be used by you without aggravating your condition. The same extends to people with a hypersensitive skin. Consult your dermatologist before you decide to use these oils in preparing laundry detergents. If they give you the green signal then go ahead with it, otherwise give it a miss.

Remember to always do a small patch test before you decide to use an essential oil for laundry or other purposes. This should include applying a little on your own skin to check for reactions and also testing on your clothes. After your detergent is done, add some to a bucket of water and soak all types of clothes for 30 minutes. Remove them and check if there is any discoloration of damage. If there isn't then it is safe to use. But if there is damage then consider using the detergent sparingly or not using it while washing the type of clothes that are damaged.

Remember that not all essential oils are suitable for laundry or aroma therapy in general. It is best that you choose one from the list mentioned in this book. You can also ask the shop keeper that you are buying it from to suggest the best type of essential oil for laundry purposes and then do some research on it to be doubly sure.

Keep the essential oils out of reach of children. Even if they accidentally come in contact with it or consume it directly, it can cause skin irritation and other such allergies. Some types of essential oils are known to induce seizures in children. They can also disturb their digestive system and burn gastrointestinal tract, so make sure to keep your children away from them. Tell them to strictly stay away from it as it is hazardous for their own health.

Remember that these are mere precautionary warnings and should not deter you from trying out making/ using essential oils for laundry purposes.

If you manage to follow the guidelines we just discussed when making laundry solution or wool dryer balls using essential oils, you will reap immense benefits of these oils in a natural manner. You will also save on a lot of money on a yearly basis.

Chapter 4: Distillation Processes

It is no secret that essential oils are extremely expensive. If you wish to use them to make a large batch then you will need quite a lot of it. If you don't fancy spending a lot of money on essential oils then it is always a good idea to make them yourself.

Now you may wonder if it is possible to make essential oils at home and the answer is, yes! It is extremely easy to extract essential oils in the very confines of your home. Let us look at 3 of the best ways in which you can extract the essential oils.

Distillation method

This is the best and easiest method and will give you the best results. You can extract as much oil as you like using this method.

To use the distillation method, you will need a distiller. A distiller is a machine that is used to extract essential oil from roots, herbs, leaves, flowers etc.

The distiller is available online and you can also check your supermarket or hardware store for one. They come in different sizes you can choose one depending on your needs.

A good distiller can cost you around $500 dollars and can be used for 10 to 12 years.

But if this price is too steep for you then you can build your own distiller. Here are the things you will need to build one.

Things required:

- 1 Standard, 10 or 15 liter, Pressure cooker
- 10 meters 10 mm Copper wire
- Water proof Sealant

- 2 inches Plastic tube
- 1 Large plastic tub
- 1 Large glass jar

Method:

➢ To build the distiller, start by cleaning the cooker thoroughly and make sure that there is no odor inside it. People prefer steel cookers to aluminum ones as aluminum can start to smell.

➢ Next, prepare the lid of the cooker. Place the copper wire over the steam valve of the lid. Use the sealant to fix the copper tubing. Make sure that there is no gap left for any steam to escape.

➢ Now insert the plastic tubing to the open end of the copper wire.

➢ Your distiller is now ready to use.

Here is how you can use the distiller.

Step 1: start by gathering all the raw materials that you will need for extracting the essential oil. This can include herbs, leaves or flowers. Let us now take lavender flowers as an example. Remember to gather both the freshest and most fragrant leaves and stalks.

Step 2: Give it a thorough wash and get rid of all dust, dirt and other impurities. You might have to clean it twice or thrice.

Step 3: Next, roughly chop them or shred using your hands and place inside the cooker. Make sure the cooker is full by 3/4ths.

Step 4: Now add in distilled water into the cooker and it should cover the lavender completely.

Step 5: Now place the lid on top of the cooker and place it on the stove. The flame should be high.

Step 6: Now, fill up the tub with cold water and place it next to the cooker. Coil the plastic tube and place it inside the cold water.

Step 7: At the end of the tubing, place a small beaker to collect the oil.

Step 8: When the cooker starts to steam, it will carry the oil with it. The tub of water will cool the steam and liquefy it.

Step 9: The beaker will collect the water that also contains the pure essential oil.

Step 10: Once the beaker is almost full you can switch off the flame and place the beaker in a cool dark place to allow the oil to settle on top of the water.

Step 11: Use a dropper to collect just the pure essential oil and place it in a small dark bottle. Make sure the bottle is sterilized.

Step 12: Place the bottle in a warm dark place for the oil to mature. It can take 24 to 48 hours for this to happen.

Your essential oil is now ready to use. You can use the same method to extract other essential oils.

Carrier oil method

The carrier oil method is the next thing that you can try. It will help you attain pure essential oil no doubt but the quality might not be as good as oil extracted through the previous method. It might not be possible to use this method for all types of oils.

To use this method, here are the things you will need.

<u>Things required:</u>

- 1 Large utensil for boiling
- 2 cups of raw materials (your choice)
- 1 cup Carrier oils such as almond or coconut

- 2 drops Vitamin E oil (buy from drugstore)
- 1 Fine cloth strainer
- 1 or 2 sterilized glass bottles

Method:

➢ Start by adding the raw materials to the large bowl along with the carrier oil and give it a good mix.
➢ Now lace it on the heat but be sure to lower the flame. You should not boil the mixture as it will fry the ingredients.
➢ Allow it to heat for 3 hours straight before switching off the heat.
➢ Allow the oil to completely cool down before running it through the fine cloth to separate the oil from the raw materials.
➢ Add in the Vitamin E oil and give it a good mix.
➢ Now transfer the concoction to a small glass bottle.
➢ Place in a warm dark place for 48 hours.
➢ Your essential oil is ready to use.

Infusion method

This is the last and probably the easiest method of all. It will give you the mildest essential oil.

Things required:

- ½ cup Carrier oil such as coconut or olive
- 1 cup raw materials (your choice, preferably flowers)
- 1 sterilized glass jar

Method:

➢ Place the raw materials in the jar and make sure there is a little space left.

- Add in the oil and close the jar tightly.
- Now shake the jar such that everything is mixed properly.
- Place the jar in a warm and dark place for 2 to 3 weeks.
- You can shake it once every week but not too much.
- You need to label all your bottles to know when they expire. Most oils last for 1 year.

These form the three ways in which you can extract essential oils from raw materials in the very confines of your home.

Chapter 5: Things To Consider When Buying Essential Oils

If you think preparing essential oils is a tedious process then buying them is the only option for you. But before you buy them, there are many things to consider in order to ensure that you are buying the right type. Here are the various things to consider while buying essential oils.

Smell

The very first thing to check is the smell of the essential oil. All essential oils will have a very strong smell and they will also be quite deep. A gentle whiff should be enough for you to get the real smell. Open the bottle and check the smell of the oil. If you think it does not smell deep enough then consider looking at other options. If you smell the presence of any other oil then don't buy it. You can also ask for some to be added to a strip of paper and smell it to see it has successfully permeated it. Once you are sure it smells concentrated, you can move to the next test.

Color

Check the color of the essential oil. Depending on what the oil is extracted from, it should have the color of the raw ingredient. So if it is an orange extract that it should be lightly orange in color, if it is lavender then it should have a light purple tinge and so on. If the colors are too vivid then it means artificial colors have been added to it. You must understand that this color might run and ruin your clothes. So it is best to buy oils that have a natural hue and there is nothing artificial.

Viscosity

Check the viscosity of the oil. A majority of the oils will be thick and will not run down easily. Use the dropper to drop a few drops into the bottle and check for thickness. If it is not thick enough then it has been diluted. Diluted ones are fine as long as the diluting agent is not used in excess of the essential oil. If it is too runny and the dropper fills up easily then don't buy it.

Names

Some essential oils will be named "fragrance oil" or "perfume oil". These are not what you want for your detergents. You have to buy something that says "pure essential oil". Check the bottle all around and make sure that these terms are not present anywhere on it. If you do spot them then don't consider them for your clothes as they will contain chemicals that will not be skin friendly.

Bottles

Remember that all essential oils are sold in dark bottles. The bottles need to be absolutely black and the contents should not be visible from the outside. If the one you are trying to buy is being sold in transparent or translucent bottles then they are definitely not pure essential oils. You must not buy them if you wish to use them for laundry purposes. Also check for a rubber or cork screw on top. Both of these will impact the flavor of the oil and so, you must not buy them. Look for screw tops instead.

Size

Remember that essential oils meant to be used for home purposes are sold in 50 ml or 100 ml quantities. If you are being sold a big bottle then it is probably excessively diluted. It is advisable to buy small bottles as you need only a little to add to your detergents. You might have a problem storing them if you buy in bulk so consider having only the small bottles and just one of each as you can use it for 3 to 4 months.

Labels

Remember to always read the labels on the bottle. If the bottle does not have any information then don't buy it. The label should tell you the country of origin, the method used for extraction, the use of any carrier oils, the ratio of dilution etc. If none of this is mentioned on the bottle then it is best to not buy it. If the bottle comes with a leaflet then read it fully buying. It might mention if the oil has been diluted. If possible, check the crop that has been used for the oil as only the best crops will produce the best oils.

Dust

Remember to check the bottles thoroughly. If you spot any dust on the top of the bottle or around the neck then it means the bottle has been sitting on the shelf for a long time. Check the date of manufacture and the expiry date. Make sure that there is at least 1 year more before the oil expires. If you think two labels have been placed each carrying different expiry dates then consider the closer one and if it is less than a year then don't buy it. If you walk home with oils that have oxidized then you will have poor quality detergents.

Method

Check the method by which the oil has been extracted. As was mentioned earlier, oils extracted by the distillation method are the best oils as they will capture a lot of the raw ingredients' essence. You can also choose the oils that have been extracted using the sponge extraction and expression methods.

Price

Always consider the price of the essential oil. The best oils will always be priced high because of their quality and long shelf life. You can expect to pay anywhere between $30 and $50 for a single bottle of essential oil. If it is being charged any lesser then it will not be pure essential oil. Don't be alarmed by the price and think of it as a long term investment. You will have the chance to use the bottle for at least 6 months if not a year. If you wish to have good quality products then you should accept the price that comes with it.

Once you buy them, remember to store them in a warm and dark place.

These are the various things to consider when you wish to buy essential oils to use for detergent and laundry purposes.

Chapter 6: Benefits of Essential Oils

By now, we have looked at the best essential oils to use for laundry, recipes to prepare them and how you can extract the essential oils by yourself.

Now, let us look at the various benefits of these essential oils and what makes them the best alternative to commercial chemical laden products.

Skin benefits

The human skin is extremely sensitive. Chemicals are capable of casing eruptions, pigmentation, drying, scaling etc. So it is important for us to use products that are not just skin friendly but also good for it. Laundry detergents contain LYE or sodium laureate sulfate and other Paraben, which can damage our skin. The best way to avoid using this chemical is by using organic soap and adding essential oils to flavor it. This will not just help protect the skin but also prevent eye redness and burning.

Aroma

It is no secret that nature puts forth some of the best aromas in the world. No chemical composition can replicate it and the scent of fresh flowers, herbs and medicinal plants is simply divine. So if you are tired of using products that contain artificial scents which start to stink after a while, it is best to shift to essential oils. Their natural aroma will tingle your senses and enliven your spirit. There are just so many smells to choose from and you can always mix and match to suit your taste. Just like you would for a perfume, you can consider using aromas based on the first note, second note and third note principle. Once you hit the winning combination, make a note of it and follow the same recipe every time that you prepare laundry detergent at home.

Anti bacterial

There are several essential oils that have an antiseptic and anti bacterial properties. These include basil, lemon, geranium, clove, tea tree etc. You can easily get rid of germs on your clothes by using these oils. Just add a few drops to the detergent and they will be good to use. You can also wipe the insides of your washing machine and dryer with tea tree oil to get rid of any germs. It is also a good idea to use this to wash your children's clothes as they would have accumulated a lot of germs while playing out in the open.

Baby clothes

It is no secret that there are not many products that cater to exclusively cleaning baby clothes. Babies have hyper sensitive skin which needs to be cared for. You cannot use commercial detergents to wash their clothes and only sterilizing them will make them dull and lifeless. The best solution is to make use of detergents prepared using essential oils. You can reduce the concentration of the oils and make a separate detergent for your baby's clothes. Using a little tea tree oil and sweet orange oil will help in keeping your baby's clothes clean and smelling sweet.

Price

Buying commercial detergents can prove to be an expensive affair. You need to buy at least 1 kilogram on a monthly basis, and that will prove to be really expensive. The best solution is to make use of essential oils to make your own detergent. You can buy organic soap in bulk and make your own essential oils. Combine the two and voila! Your detergent is ready to use. You can store the detergent for up to 6 months or more and will depend on the expiry date of the essential oil. You need to label them to know by when they need to be used.

Environment

Everybody is now environment conscious. If you wish to give your children a greener future, then consider abandoning chemical laden products. This includes store bought detergents. The water that is used while washing your clothes is sent back to nature. They will contain the chemicals present in your detergent and cause out environment harm. The best way to solve this problem is by using essential oils and you will end up giving back to Earth, its own natural produce. This will help in cleaning the environment and by not using plastics you will reduce your carbon foot prints.

Chapter 7: Homemade Laundry Detergent Recipes With Essential Oils

Homemade Laundry Detergent Powder for Whitening

Materials Required:

- 1 cup borax
- 2 cups laundry soap flakes or grate laundry soap
- 1 cup washing soda
- 2 cups baking soda
- 2 tablespoons lemon essential oil

Procedure:

1. Mix together all the ingredients well and store in an airtight plastic container.
2. Label the container with usage instructions.
3. Use ½ cup for every wash load.

Floral Homemade Laundry Detergent Powder

Materials Required:

- 1 cup borax
- 2 cups laundry soap flakes or grate laundry soap
- 1 cup washing soda
- 2 cups baking soda
- 2 tablespoons lavender essential oil
- 1 tablespoon rosemary essential oil.

Procedure:

1. Mix together all the ingredients well and store in an airtight plastic container.
2. Label the container with usage instructions.
3. Use ½ cup for every wash load.

Fruity Homemade Laundry Detergent Powder

Materials Required:

- 1 cup borax
- 2 cups laundry soap flakes or grate laundry soap
- 1 cup washing soda
- 2 cups baking soda
- 2 tablespoons geranium essential oil
- 2 tablespoons sweet orange essential oil.

Procedure:

1. Mix together all the ingredients well and store in an airtight plastic container. Label the container with usage instructions.
2. Use ½ cup for every wash load.

Laundry Detergent powder with zote

Materials:

- 2 bars zote soap (14 ounce each), chopped into 1 – 2 inch pieces
- 6 cups borax
- 6 cups washing soda
- 20 drops lime essential oil
- 20 drops orange essential oil

- 20 drops vanilla essential oil

Procedure:

1. Using a food processor, grate the zote soap into fine granules.
2. Add borax, washing soda and essential oil.
3. Store in an air tight container.
4. Label the container with usage instructions.
5. Use 1 to 2 tablespoons per wash load.

Eco Friendly All natural Laundry Detergent

Materials required:

- 1 cup borax
- 1 cup baking soda
- 1 cup Epsom salt
- 1 ½ bars pure castile soap, grated
- 10 drops tea tree oil

Procedure:

1. Place the castile soap in a blender and powder it.
2. Remove from the blender. Mix together borax, baking sodas, Epsom salt, powdered castile soap and tea tree oil.
3. Transfer to an air tight container.
4. Label the container with usage instructions.
5. Use a tablespoon of the detergent for small loads or 2 tablespoons for large loads.

Natural Wash & Stain Remover Bar Soap:

Materials required:

- 21.6 ounce coconut oil (that has a melting point of 76 degrees)
- 36 ounce palm oil
- 14.4 ounce soya bean oil
- 10.4 ounce lye
- 22 ounce water
- 1.5 ounce borax
- 20 drops sweet orange essential oil
- 0.8 ounce lemon essential oil
- Soap molds

- Thermometer
- Parchment paper
- Hand gloves
- Glasses to cover your eyes

Procedure:

1. Take a large ceramic or glass container. Add water to it.
2. Slowly add lye to the water in the container stirring constantly. (Do not add water to lye)
3. Mix well and set aside to cool.
4. Meanwhile place coconut oil and palm oil in a sauce pan. Heat the saucepan until the oil reaches a temperature of 120 – 130 degree F.
5. Transfer the coconut oil mixture to a crock pot. Add soya bean oil. Set the crock pot on low.
6. Gently pour the lye mixture to the crock pot. Mix well a couple of times.
7. Use a stick blender and blend until smooth and thick. Cover and cook for about 45 minutes. The mixture in the pot should be rising up and folding back.
8. When your soap is ready, it will be slightly translucent. Check by dipping a ph. strip in the soap. If the soap is done, the ph. value should be in between 7 -10. Add borax and stir well.
9. Let the mixture cool for a while.
10.   Add the essential oils at this stage else the fragrance will be lost.
11.   Line soap molds with parchment paper. Pour the soap into the molds.
12.   Let it cool. Remove from the molds and cut into desired size.

Laundry Detergent with oxyclean

Materials required:

- 3 cups borax
- 1 1/3 cups washing soda
- 2 containers (3 pounds each) oxyclean
- 4 bars zote soap, grated
- 3 cups baking soda
- 4 bottles crystal fabric enhancer
- 30 drops of orange essential oil
- 30 drops of grapefruit essential oil
- 30 drops of lemongrass or lime essential oil

Procedure:

1. Mix together all the ingredients in a large bucket.
2. Store in an air tight container.
3. Label the container with usage instructions.
4. Use about ¼ cup per laundry load.

Pure Coconut oil Laundry Soap

Materials required:

- 66 ounce coconut oil (that has a melting point of 76 degrees)
- 11.8 ounce lye
- 24 ounce water
- 2 ounce lavender oil
- Soap molds
- Thermometer
- Parchment paper
- Hand gloves
- Glasses to cover your eyes

Procedure:

1. Take a large ceramic or glass container. Add water to it.

2. Slowly add lye to the water in the container stirring constantly. (Do not add water to lye)
3. Mix well and set aside to cool.
4. Meanwhile place coconut oil in a sauce pan. Heat the saucepan until the oil reaches a temperature of 120 – 130 degree F.
5. Transfer the coconut oil to a crock pot. Set the crock pot on low.
6. Gently pour the lye mixture to the crock pot. Mix well a couple of times.
7. Use a stick blender and blend until smooth and thick. Cover and cook for about 45 minutes. The mixture in the pot should be rising up and folding back.
8. When your soap is ready, it will be slightly translucent. Check by dipping a ph. strip in the soap. If the soap is done, the ph. value should be in between 7 -10.
9. Let the mixture cool for a while.
10.   Add the essential oils at this stage else the fragrance will be lost.
11.   Line soap molds with parchment paper. Pour the soap into the molds.
12.   Let it cool. Remove from the molds and cut into desired size.

Laundry Detergent for Hard water

Materials required:

- 2 bars fels Naptha, finely grated
- 2 cups washing soda
- 2 cups borax
- 25-30 drops essential oils of your choice
- 7 cups water

Procedure:

1. Add fels Naptha to water and melt it. Remove from heat.
2. Add borax and washing soda.
3. Mix well. Transfer into a big jar with a lid and store. Label the container with usage instructions.
4. Use 1 – 1 ½ tablespoons per load of clothes.

Stain Fighting Laundry Detergent

Materials Required:

- 1 cup borax
- 1 cup laundry soap flakes or grate laundry soap
- 1 cup washing soda
- 1 bar Fels Naptha, grated
- 10 drops tea tree essential oil

Procedure:

1. Place all the ingredients in a food processor. Pulse until it is mixed well.
2. Store in an airtight plastic container. Label the container with usage instructions.
3. Use 1 tablespoon for a regular wash load.
4. For dirty clothes or larger loads, use 2-3 tablespoons.
5. For top loading washing machine, fill the machine with a couple of liters of water. Add the detergent so as to dissolve.

Low Suds Powder

Materials Required:

- 2 cups borax
- 2 cups laundry soap flakes or grate laundry soap
- 2 cups washing soda
- 20 – 30 drops essential oils of your choice

Procedure:

1. Place all the ingredients in a food processor. Pulse until it is mixed well.
2. Store in an airtight plastic container.
3. Label the container with usage instructions.
4. Use 1 tablespoon for a regular wash load.
5. For dirty clothes or larger loads, use 2-3 tablespoons.
6. For top loading washing machine, fill the machine with a couple of liters of water. Add the detergent so as to dissolve.

High Efficiency (HE) Detergent Powder -1

Materials Required:

- 2 cups borax
- 2 bars grated laundry soap
- 2 cups washing soda
- 30 drops of orange essential oil
- 30 drops of grapefruit essential oil
- 30 drops of lemongrass or lime essential oil
- 2 cups oxygen booster

Procedure:

1. Place all the ingredients in a food processor. Pulse until it is mixed well.
2. Store in an airtight plastic container. Label the container with usage instructions.
3. Use 1 tablespoon for a regular wash load.
4. For dirty clothes or larger loads, use 2-3 tablespoons.
5. For top loading washing machine, fill the machine with a couple of liters of water. Add the detergent so as to dissolve.

High Efficiency (HE) Detergent Powder -2

Materials required:

- 6 bars fels Naptha, grated
- 15 ounce borax
- 110 ounce washing soda
- 4 cups baking soda
- 4 containers oxyclean
- 4 containers fabric softener crystals

Procedure:

1. Mix all the ingredients together.
2. Put them in a large airtight container. Label the container with usage instructions.
3. Use 2 tablespoon per normal load. Put it directly into the tub and not into the dispenser.

Laundry Detergent Balls

Materials Required:

- 4 cups baking soda
- 2 cups borax
- 4 cups clear glycerin soap flakes or grate glycerin soap
- 1 teaspoon chamomile essential oil

Procedure:

1. Mix together all the ingredients well.
2. Make small balls of about an inch diameter.
3. Store in an airtight plastic container. Label the container with usage instructions.
4. Use 1 ball for every wash load.
5. Use within 2 months.

Chapter 8: Homemade Liquid Laundry Detergent Recipes With Essential Oils

Homemade Liquid Laundry Detergent using stove -1

Materials Required:

- 2 cups borax
- 2 cups laundry bar soap (grated)
- 2 cups washing soda
- 4 cups boiling water
- 4 gallons tepid water
- 2 tablespoons of lavender essential

Procedure:

1. Boil water on low heat.
2. Add the grated soap bar slowly and keep stirring till it has completely melted and there are no lumps left. Let it cool over night
3. Add lavender essential oil.
4. Pour the liquid mixture into a large bucket (make sure it is pretty big)
5. Gently add borax and washing soda.
6. Add 4 gallons of water and mix the whole concoction till everything is uniform.
7. Store in large jars or bottles with lids. Label the container with usage instructions.
8. Use ¼th cup for every wash load. Stir the mixture before using it as it can start to set.

Liquid Laundry Detergent Recipe without Using Stove

Materials Required:

- 4 ounce liquid castile soap
- 4 tablespoons glycerin
- 4 cups washing soda
- 4 cups baking soda
- 8 cups warm water
- 20 drops eucalyptus essential oil

Procedure:

1. Mix together all the ingredients well and store in an airtight plastic container. Label the container with usage instructions.
2. Use ¼ cup for every wash load.

Liquid Homemade Laundry Detergent using stove- 2

Materials Required:

- ½ cup borax
- 2 laundry bar soap (grated)
- 2 cups washing soda
- 8 cups boiling water
- 1 tablespoon lemon essential oil
- 1 tablespoon of lavender essential
- 1 tablespoon clove essential oil

Procedure:

1. Boil water on low heat.
2. Add the grated soap bar slowly and keep stirring till it has completely melted and there are no lumps left.
3. Pour the liquid mixture into a large bucket.
4. Gently add borax and washing soda.

5. Stir well. Let it cool overnight.
6. Add the essential oils
7. Store in large jars or bottles with lids. Label the container with usage instructions.
8. Use 1 cup for every top load wash load. Stir the mixture before using it as it can start to set.
9. Use ½ a cup for front load wash.
10. Use ¼ cup for every wash load.

Lemon scented Liquid Homemade Laundry Detergent

Materials Required:

- 2 laundry bar soap (grated)
- 4 cups baking soda
- 4 gallons boiling water
- 1 tablespoon lemon essential oil

Procedure:

1. Boil water just enough to cover the grated soap on low heat.
2. Add the grated soap bar slowly and keep stirring till it has completely melted and there are no lumps left.
3. Pour the liquid mixture into a large bucket. Add 4 gallons boiling water and stir well.
4. Add baking soda and mix well.
5. Add essential oil and mix well.
6. Store in large jars or bottles with lids. Label the container with usage instructions.
7. Use ½ cup for a normal load. Use more for dirtier or larger load.

Minty Homemade Liquid Laundry Detergent

Materials Required:

- 2 laundry bar soap (grated)
- 4 cups baking soda
- 4 gallons boiling water
- 1 teaspoon mint essential oil
- 1 teaspoon eucalyptus essential oil

Procedure:

1 Boil water just enough to cover the grated soap on low heat.
2 Add the grated soap bar slowly and keep stirring till it has completely melted and there are no lumps left.
3 Pour the liquid mixture into a large bucket. Add 4 gallons boiling water and stir well.
4 Add baking soda and mix well.
5 Add essential oil and mix well.
6 Store in large jars or bottles with lids. Label the container with usage instructions.
7 Use ½ cup for a normal load. Use more for dirtier or larger load.

Lavender Chamomile Liquid Homemade Laundry Detergent

Materials Required:

- 1 cup borax

- 2/3 bar Fels Naptha, grated
- 1 cup washing soda
- 12 cups boiling water
- 4 tablespoons glycerin
- 1 tablespoon of lavender essential oil
- 1 tablespoon chamomile essential oil

Procedure

1. Mix together grated soap and 12 cups hot water and place on low heat. Keep stirring till it has completely melted and there are no lumps left.
2. Add washing soda and borax. Stir constantly until the mixture thickens.
3. Remove from heat.
4. Pour the liquid mixture into a large bucket.
5. Add 2 quarts of hot water to the bucket.
6. Stir well. Add glycerin. Let it cool for 24 hours.
7. Add the essential oils.
8. Add 2 – 3 cups of hot water. Stir well.
9. Store in large jars or bottles with lids. Label the container with usage instructions.
10. Use 1 cup for every top load wash load. Stir the mixture before using it as it can start to set.
11. Use ½ a cup for front load wash.
12. Use ¼ cup for every wash load.

Liquid Homemade Laundry Detergent - 4

Materials Required:

- 1 cup washing soda

- ½ cup baking soda
- ½ cup Celtic sea salt or Epsom salt
- 2 cups liquid castile soap
- 2 tablespoons house hold cleaner (optional)
- 20 drops chamomile essential drops

Procedure:

1. Add about 8 cups water to a large pot and bring to a boil.
2. Slowly add washing soda, baking soda and salt. Mix well until completely dissolved
3. Cool and transfer into a bucket with a tight lid.
4. Add 2 more cups of water, house hold cleaner and essential oil. Stir well and close the lid.
5. Stir well before using the detergent. Label the container with usage instructions.
6. Add ½ cup to a regular load of clothes and add more for soiled clothes.

Liquid Laundry Soap – 5

Materials required:

- 2 bars (14 ounce each) zote laundry soap
- 4 cups borax
- 4 cups washing soda
- Water as required
- 20 drops juniper essential oil

Procedure:

1. Take a large pot or a large container. Add zote soap to the container.

2. Add about 4 quarts water and place the container over medium heat. Let it simmer for about 45 minutes or until the soap melts.
3. Add 4 quarts of water and simmer
4. Add 2 more quarts water and bring to a simmer. Add borax and washing soda. Mix well until completely dissolved.
5. Remove from heat and transfer to a large 10 gallon bucket. Fill up the bucket with water and mix well.
6. Transfer this soap into wide mouthed containers or jars. Label the container with usage instructions.
7. To use, melt about ½ a cup of the soap concentrate and add it to 1 ½ cups water. Mix well and use.

Homemade Laundry Soap with Dish Soap

Materials required:

- 2/3 cup washing soda
- ½ cup borax
- ¼ cup dish soap
- 2 gallons tap water

Procedure:

1. Fill a bucket with half a gallon of boiling hot water.
2. Add washing soda and borax.
3. Mix well until the borax and washing soda is completely dissolved.
4. Add dish soap. Mix well. Add 2 gallons of tap water gently. Mix well.
5. Store in large jars with lids on it. Label the container with usage instructions.
6. Remember this soap is a thin liquid soap.
7. Use about ½ to ¾ cup per load of clothes.

Chapter 9: Laundry Detergent Recipes Without Borax

Laundry Detergent without Borax - 1

Materials required:

- 2 bars finely grated glycerin soap
- 1 cup baking soda
- 2 cups washing sod
- 1 cup citric acid
- ½ cup rock salt

Procedure:

1. Mix together all the ingredients well and store in an airtight plastic container. Label the container with usage instructions.
2. Use 1- 2 tablespoons for every wash load.

Laundry Detergent without Borax – 2

Materials required:

- 8 cups baking soda
- 6 cups washing sod
- 4 cups castile soap, grated
- 10 drops lavender essential oil

Procedure:

1. Mix together all the ingredients well and store in an airtight plastic container. Label the container with usage instructions.

2. Use 1- 2 tablespoons for every wash load.

Laundry liquid detergent without borax -1

Materials required:

- 1 liter castile soap
- 30 drops lavender essential oil
- 20 drops lemon essential oil
- 20 drops orange essential

Procedure:

1. Add all the ingredients to a large bottle. Shake well and store. Label the container with usage instructions.
2. Use 1/3 cup for a normal load.

Lemony liquid detergent without borax -2

Materials required:

- 1 liter castile soap
- 10 drops lemon grass essential oil
- 20 drops lemon essential oil
- 10 drops chamomile essential oil

Procedure:

1. Add all the ingredients to a large bottle. Shake well and store. Label the container with usage instructions.
2. Use 1/3 cup for a normal load.

Chapter 10: Detergent Recipes With Essential Oils For Cloth Diapers

All-natural Cloth Diaper Detergent

Materials required:

- 1 cup Epsom salt
- 1 cup washing soda
- 1 cup baking soda
- 1 cup baby oxyclean
- 20 drops of tea tree essential oil
- 15 drops of lemongrass or lemon essential oil
- 10 drops of Palmarosa essential oil

Procedure:

1. Mix together all the ingredients in a food processor. Pulse until well combined.
2. Store in an air tight container. Label the container with usage instructions.
3. Add 1 tablespoon for a normal load. Add more for dirty clothes or larger loads.
4. Note: Use more Epsom salt if the water is hard while making the detergent.

Detergent for Cloth Diapers

Materials required:

- 2 cups washing soda
- 2 cups borax

- 1 cup oxyclean
- 20 drops oregano essential oil
- 20 drops orange essential oil

Procedure:

1. Mix together all the ingredients well and store in an airtight plastic container. Label the container with usage instructions.
2. Use 1 – 2 tablespoons for every wash load.

Stain Remover Detergent for Cloth Diapers

Materials required:

- 4 cups washing soda
- 2 cups baking soda
- 2 cups baby oxyclean
- 20 drops of tea tree essential oil
- 15 drops of orange essential oil

Procedure:

1. Mix together all the ingredients well and store in an airtight plastic container. Label the container with usage instructions.
2. Use 1 – 2 tablespoons for every wash load.

Chapter 11: Recipes For Fabric Softeners With Essential Oils

Naturally Scented Fabric Softener

Materials required:

- 4 cups Epsom salt or course sea salt
- 20 drops of lavender
- 15 drops of lemongrass or lemon
- 10 drops of clove essential oil
- 1 cup baking soda

Procedure:

1. Mix together Epsom salt and essential oils.
2. Add baking soda and mix well.
3. Store in an air tight container. Label the container with usage instructions.
4. Add 1 – 2 tablespoons to the clothes just before rinsing.

Tea tree Scented Fabric Softener

Materials required:

- 6 cups white vinegar
- ½ cup rubbing alcohol or vodka
- 30 drops tea tree essential oil

. **Procedure:**

1. Place together all the ingredients in a large jar or bottle with a tight fitting cap, Shake well and use. Label the container with usage instructions.
2. Add ½ to ¾ cup to the fabric softener dispenser in the washing machine

Homemade Fabric Softener with Conditioner-1

Materials required:

- 3 Cups Water
- 1 cups hair conditioner
- 1 ½ Cups White Vinegar
- 10 drops of orange essential oil
- 10 drops of grapefruit essential oil
- 10 drops of lemongrass or lime essential oil

Procedure:

1. Place together all the ingredients in a large jar or bottle with a tight fitting cap, Shake well and use. Label the container with usage instructions.
2. Add ½ to ¾ cup to the fabric softener dispenser in the washing machine

Fabric Softener

Materials required:

- 1 ½ Cups White Vinegar
- 5 drops lavender essential oil

Procedure:

1. Place together all the ingredients in a large jar or bottle with a tight fitting cap, Shake well and use. Label the container with usage instructions.
2. Add ½ cup to the rinse cycle

Fabric Softener with Baking soda

Materials required:

- 1 ½ Cups White Vinegar
- 5 drops chamomile essential oil
- 3 cups hot water
- 1 ½ cups baking soda

Procedure:

1. Add water and baking soda in a bucket. Mix well.
2. Slowly pour the vinegar into the bucket. It will start fizzing. Once the fizz becomes flat, store in a large bottle. Label the container with usage instructions.
3. Shake well before each use.
4. Use ¼ cup in the rinse cycle.

Fabric Softener Recipe for Dryer

Materials required:

- ½ cup baking soda

- 4 teaspoons cornstarch (optional)
- 6 drops lavender essential oil

Procedure:

1. Mix together baking soda and corn starch.
2. Add essential oils. Mix well.
3. Store in an airtight container. Label the container with usage instructions.
4. To use: Make a small pouch using sheer fabric. Add 1 tablespoon of the softener into the bag. Seal it with a string or rubber band and place it in the dryer.

Chapter 12: Laundry Starch Recipes With Essential Oils

Laundry Starch Recipe -1

Materials required:

- 3 tablespoons corn starch
- 5 cups water
- 10 drops lemon essential oil

Procedure:

1. Mix together cornstarch and water. Bring to a boil. Cool down completely.
2. Pour into a spray bottle. Add essential oil. Shake well before use. Label the container with usage instructions.
3. Spray on the desired fabric.

Laundry Starch Recipe -2

Materials required:

- 2/3 cup vodka
- 1 1/3 cup water
- 10 drops orange essential oil

Procedure:

1. Mix together vodka and water and pour into a spray bottle.

2. Add essential oil. Shake well and use. Label the container with usage instructions.

Chapter 13: Laundry Detergent Recipes for Wool

Homemade Wool Wash - 1

Materials required:

- 8 cups soap flakes
- 8 cups boiling water
- 2 cups denatured alcohol
- 1 tablespoon lavender essential oil
- 1 tablespoon eucalyptus essential oil

Procedure:

1. Add soap flakes and boiling water to a bowl.
2. Using a stick blender, whisk the mixture well.
3. Add denatured alcohol and essential oils. Mix well.
4. Transfer to a large jar with a lid. Let it set overnight. Close the lid and store. Label the container with usage instructions.
5. To use, add a tablespoon of the detergent to Luke warm water. Soak the woolens in it for a while and rinse.

Homemade Wool Wash – 2

Materials required:

- 4 cups soap flakes
- 8 cups boiling water
- 13 ounce denatured alcohol
- 4 ounce eucalyptus oil

Procedure:

Essential Oils

1. Mix together all the ingredients.
2. Store in a container. Label the container with usage instructions.
3. To use, add 1 to 2 tablespoons to a cup of hot water, Mix well until it dissolves completely. Add it to Luke warm water, Soak woolens in it for a while and rinse.

Homemade Wool Wash – 3

Materials required:

- 2 cups hot water
- ½ teaspoon lanolin
- ½ teaspoon baby shampoo
- 5 drops rose essential drops
- 2 cups hot water

Procedure:

1. Mix together all the ingredients, Mix well until the lanolin has dissolved.
2. Add this to Luke warm water. Soak your woolens in this solution and rinse well.
3. Best suited for hand washed woolens.

Homemade Wool Wash – 4

Materials required:

- 1 teaspoon shampoo
- 2 teaspoons fels Naptha soap, grated
- 2 teaspoons liquid castile soap

Procedure:

1. Mix together all the ingredients and store in a bottle.
2. Use ¼ teaspoon of this in half a bucket of Luke warm water.
3. Soak your woolens in this solution and rinse well.
4. Best suited for hand washed woolens

Conclusion

I want to thank you once again for choosing this book. In this book we learnt how essential oils can be used with organic laundry solutions instead of chemical laced laundry products, which can cause skin infection or ruin the thread of your clothes. From cleaning laundry to softening them, essential oils can be used in many areas.

Another good way to incorporate essential oils in your laundry is by using them with wool dryer balls. These balls originated as a way to replace the synthetic dryer sheets in use. In combination with essential oils, wool dryer balls work efficiently and the clothes remain fresh and fragrant for a longer time.

Essential oils might appear as a costly affair as they are priced high for very small quantities. Their extraction and raw material makes them costly. But the point to be noted here is that essential oils are available in concentrated forms. They have to be used in diluted forms. So long as you apply essential oils in the right form and right quantity, they can do wonders with your laundry.

So without much ado, get started on making your very own organic or chemical free laundry solutions and reap the benefits of essential oils and organic cleaning products.

www.ingramcontent.com/pod-product-compliance
Lightning Source LLC
Chambersburg PA
CBHW070813290526

45795CB00002B/703